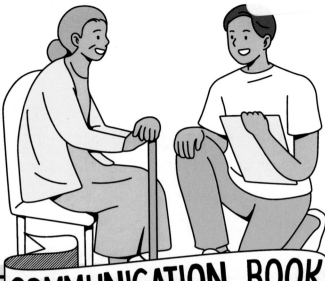

COMMUNICATION BOOK

THIS BOOK BELONGS TO:

_____

_____

_____

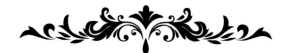

How to Use This Book?

Understanding Non-Verbal Communication Cards

Non-verbal communication cards, often referred to as Picture Exchange Communication Systems (PECS), comprise a set of visual aids featuring images or symbols representing various concepts, actions, and objects. These cards typically feature simple images or symbols representing common needs, emotions, or everyday activities. For elderly individuals with conditions such as aphasia, dementia, or the aftereffects of a stroke, these cards offer an invaluable means of expression.

Who Can Benefit from Non-Verbal Communication Cards

- Adults or seniors with temporary or long term speech loss and unable to speak.
- Adults or seniors who need help with personal care due to stroke, brain injury, intubation, ALS, cerebral palsy, dementia, aphasia, Down Syndrome and IDD.
- Adults or seniors with autism or related conditions.
- Caregivers, educators, family, health care and hospice professionals who work with nonverbal individuals.

Benefits of Non-Verbal Communication Cards

- Facilitating expression.
- Reducing frustration caused by misunderstandings.
- Promoting independence, enhance their sense of autonomy and dignity, which is especially important for maintaining their mental well-being.

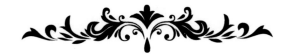

- Supporting memory and cognition.
- Enhancing caregiver-patient interaction, as caregivers can more accurately interpret and address the patient's needs.

How to Use Non-Verbal Communication Cards

1. Introduction and Familiarization: Introduce the individual each picture of this book, ensuring they understand the meaning of each symbol or image. Simply point to the pictures using a finger or stylus to indicate a choice.

2. Practice and Reinforcement: Engage in regular practice sessions to reinforce the use of these pictures. Encourage them to select which symbol to express their needs, desires, or emotions.

3. Integration into Daily Routine: Incorporate this book into daily activities and routines. Use them during meal times, transitions, and social interactions to promote consistent usage.

4. Individualized Approach: Tailor the selection of non-verbal communication cards to the their preferences and needs. There are blank templates provided in this book to customize the board with personal favorite pictures or words.

5. Encouragement and Positive Reinforcement: Give praise and encouragement for using non-verbal communication cards effectively. Reinforce their efforts with positive feedback to motivate continued progress.

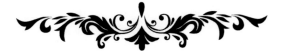

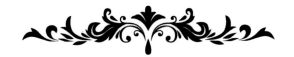

Tips for Effective Communication

- Patience and Understanding: Approach communication with patience and empathy, understanding each individual with ASD may require additional time to process information and respond.

- Respect Personal Space: Respect the individual's personal space and boundaries, allowing them to communicate at their own pace and comfort level.

- Clear and Simple Language: When using verbal communication alongside non-verbal communication cards, employ clear and simple language to enhance comprehension.

- Use Visual Cues: Incorporate visual cues and gestures to supplement verbal and non-verbal communication, providing additional support and context.

- Encourage Self-Advocacy: Foster self-advocacy skills by encouraging the individual to initiate communication using non-verbal communication cards and advocate for their needs and preferences.

Feelings

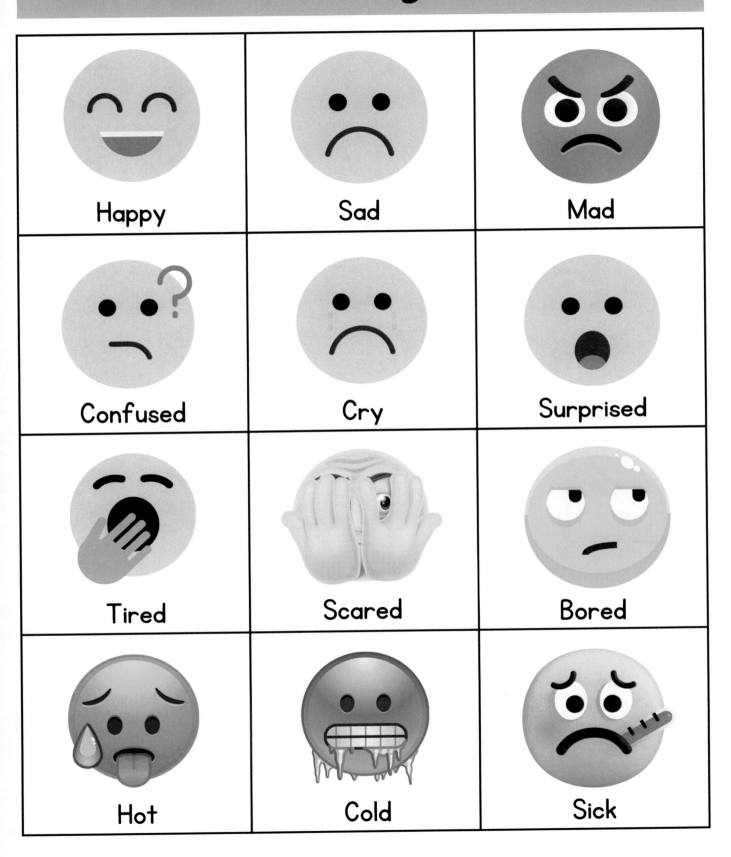

Happy	Sad	Mad
Confused	Cry	Surprised
Tired	Scared	Bored
Hot	Cold	Sick

Communication

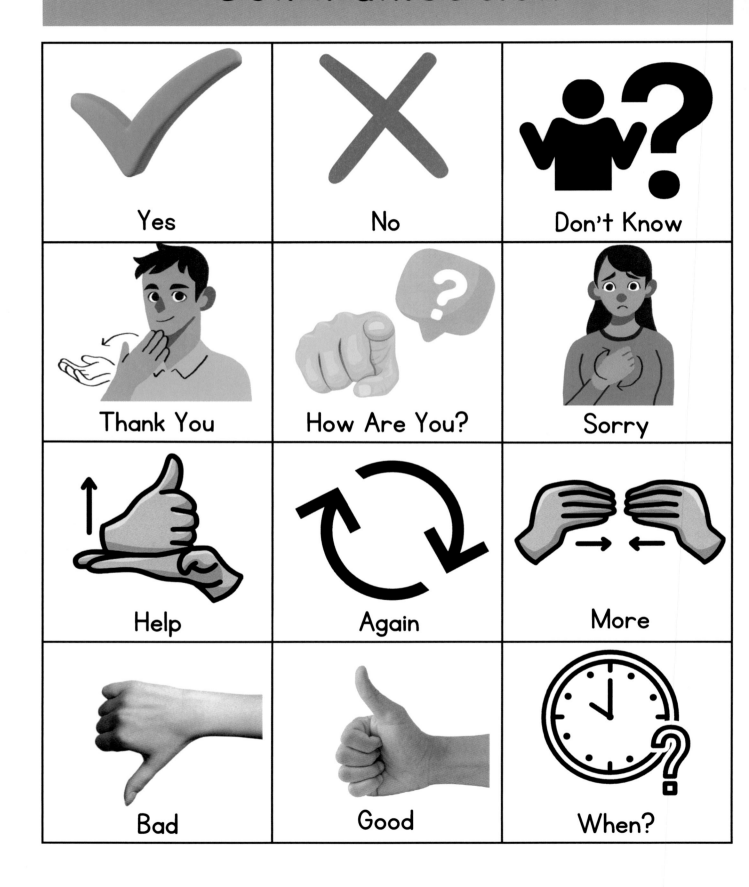

Yes	No	Don't Know
Thank You	How Are You?	Sorry
Help	Again	More
Bad	Good	When?

Communication

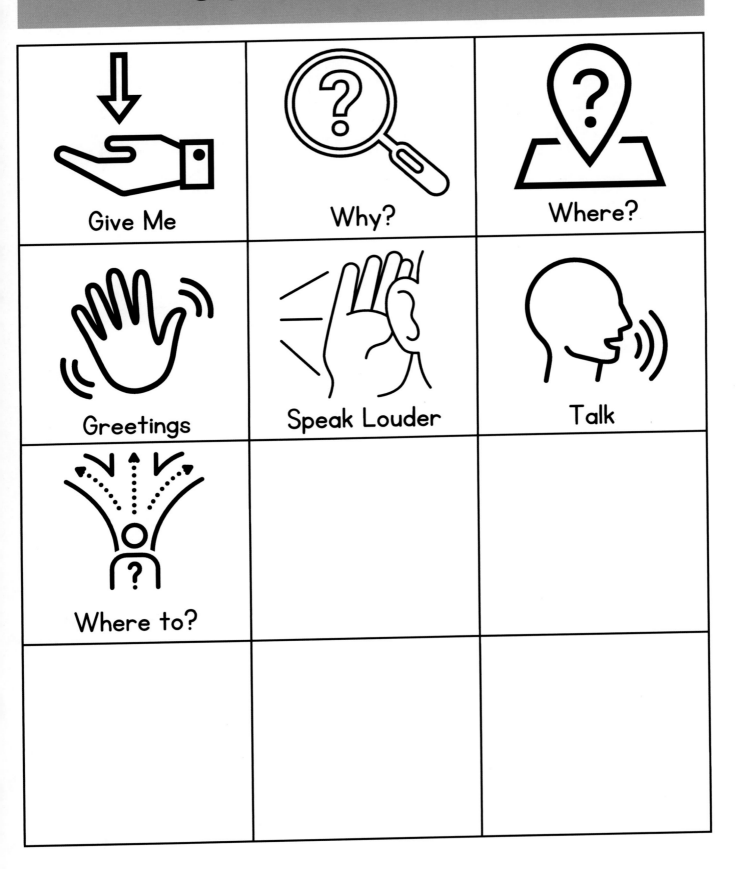

Give Me	Why?	Where?
Greetings	Speak Louder	Talk
Where to?		

Bathing

Change

You

No

I need

More

Help

Done

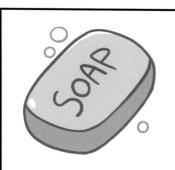 Soap	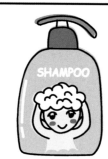 Shampoo	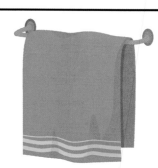 Towel
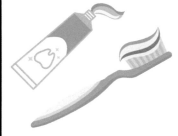 Brush Teeth	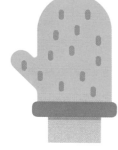 Washcloth	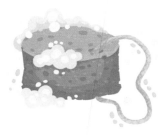 Scrub
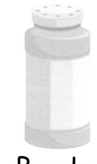 Powder	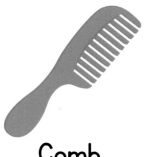 Comb	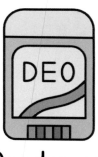 Deodorant
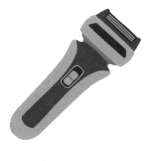 Shaver	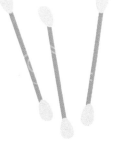 Q-Tips	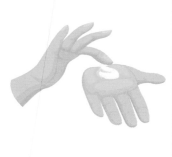 Lotion

Dressing

I need		

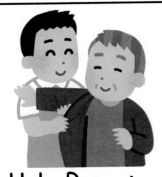
Help Dressing

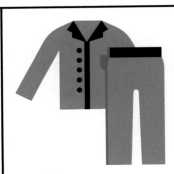
Pajamas

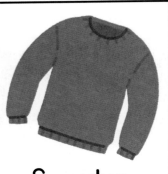
Sweater

You

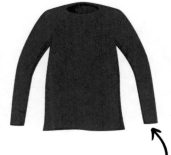
Long Sleeve Shirt

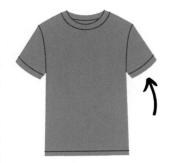
Short Sleeve Shirt

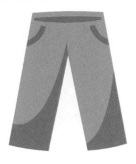
Long Pants

No

Change

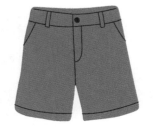
Short Pants

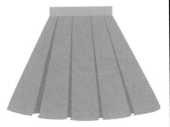
Skirt

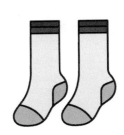
Socks

More

Help

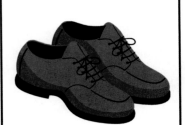
Shoes

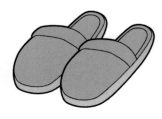
Slippers

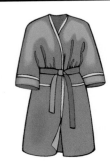
Robe

Done

Meal Time

I'm

You

No

I need

More

Help

Done

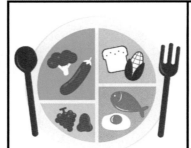Food	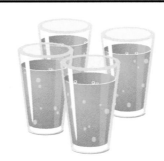Drink	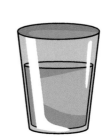Water
Hungry	Not Hungry	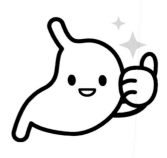Full
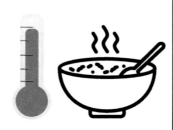Too Hot	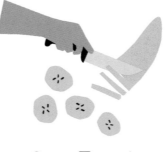Cut Food	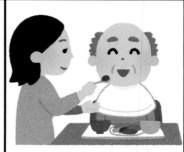Help Eat
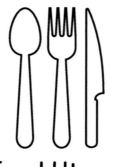Food Utensils	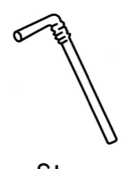Straw	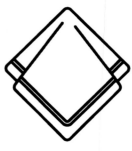Napkin

Food

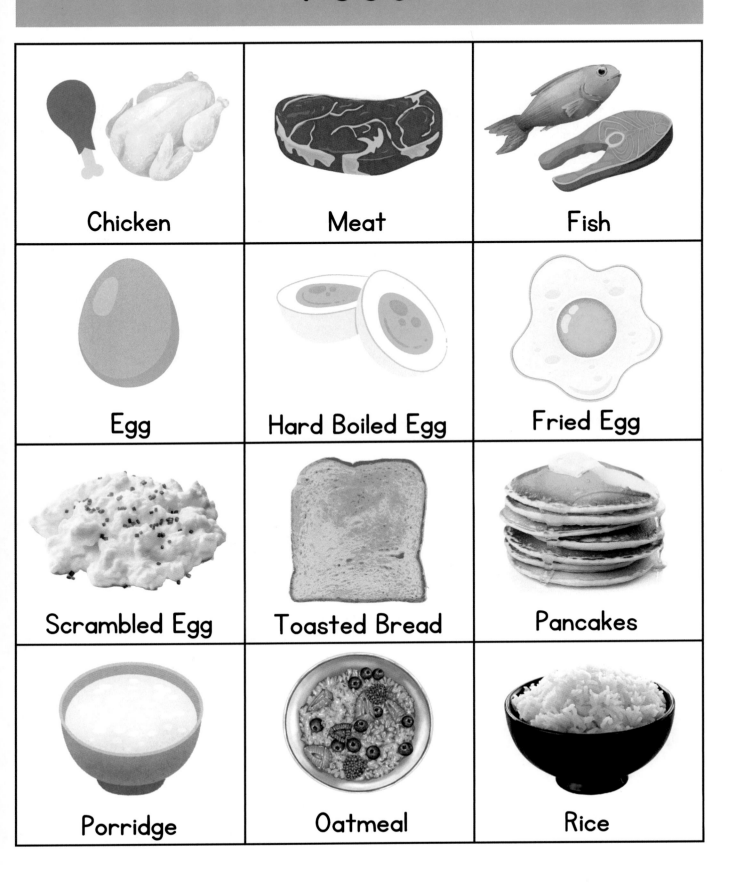

Chicken	Meat	Fish
Egg	Hard Boiled Egg	Fried Egg
Scrambled Egg	Toasted Bread	Pancakes
Porridge	Oatmeal	Rice

Food

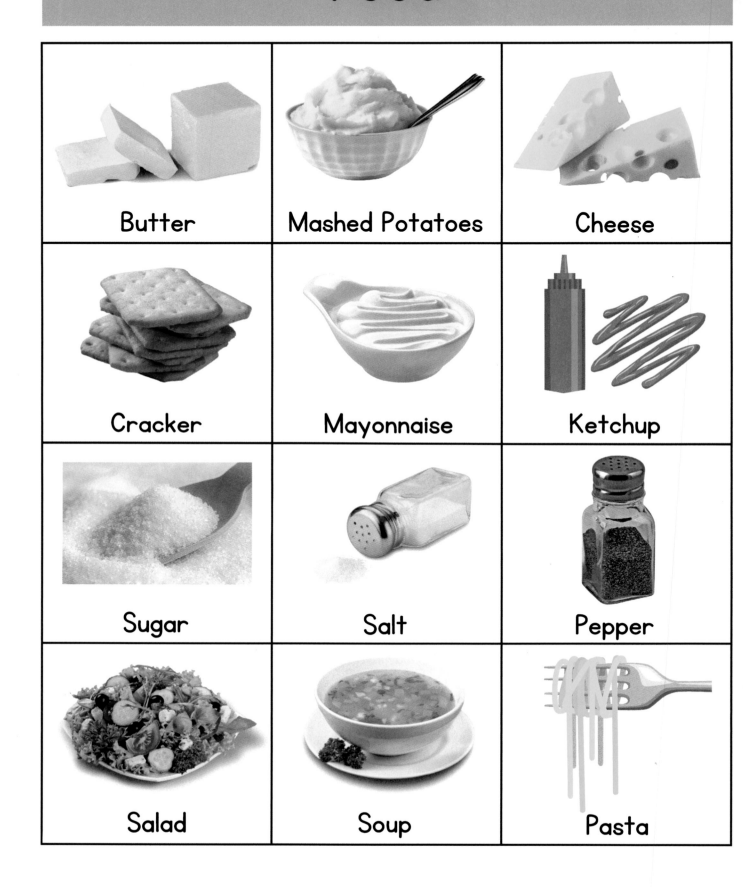

Butter	Mashed Potatoes	Cheese
Cracker	Mayonnaise	Ketchup
Sugar	Salt	Pepper
Salad	Soup	Pasta

Fruits

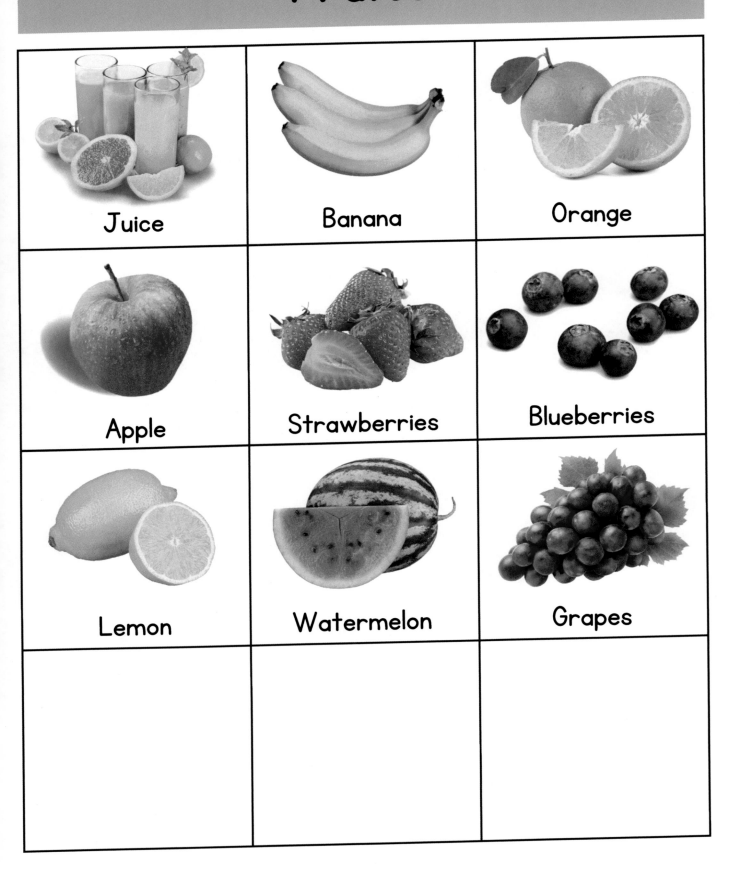

Juice	Banana	Orange
Apple	Strawberries	Blueberries
Lemon	Watermelon	Grapes

Drinks

Water	Tea	Coffee
Protein Shakes	Milk	Kombucha

Pain Scale

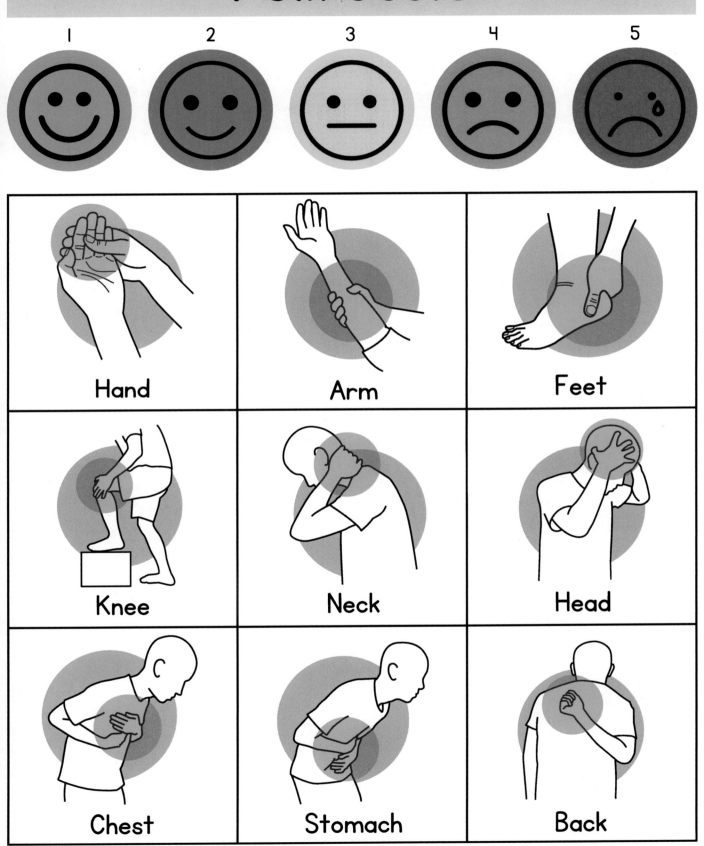

Medical

I need			
You	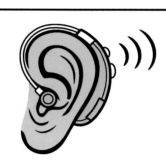 Hearing Aid	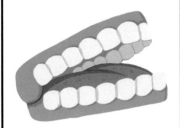 Dentures	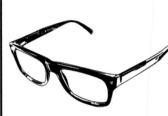 Glasses
No			
Change	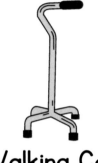 Walking Cane	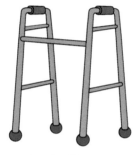 Walker	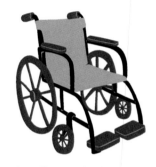 Wheelchair
More	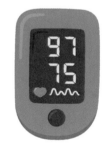 Pulse Oximeter	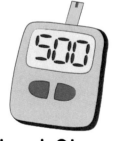 Blood Glucose Monitor	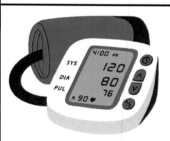 Blood Pressure Monitor
Help			
Done	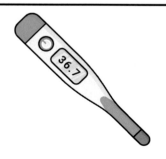 Thermometer	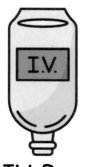 IV Bag	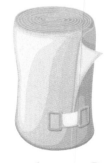 Bandage Roll

Medical

Change
You
No
I need
More
Help
Done

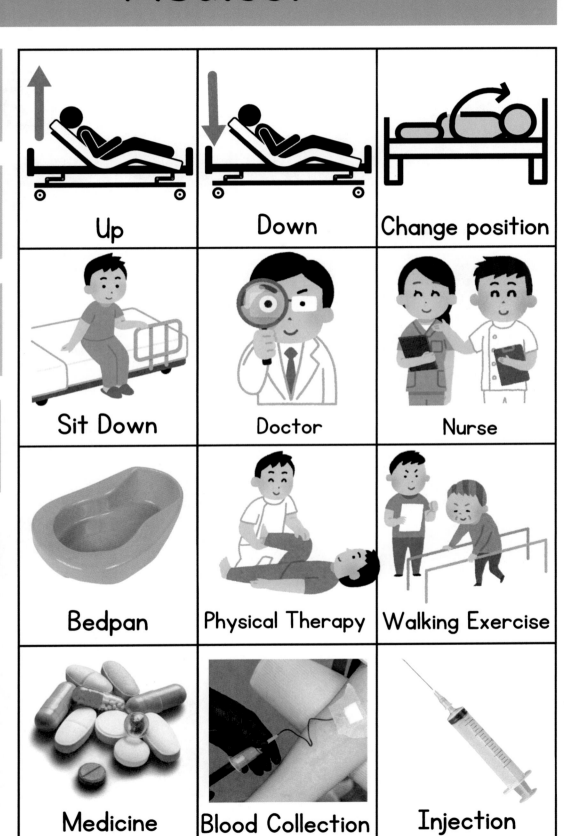

Up	Down	Change position
Sit Down	Doctor	Nurse
Bedpan	Physical Therapy	Walking Exercise
Medicine	Blood Collection	Injection

Activities

I want			
You	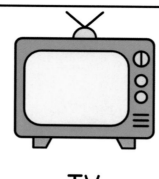 TV	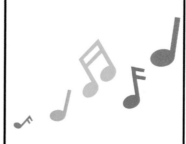 Music	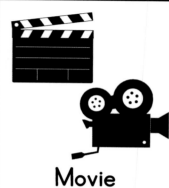 Movie
No	 Read	Play Chess	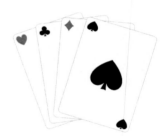 Card Game
Change			
More	Puzzle	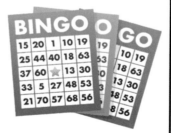 Bingo	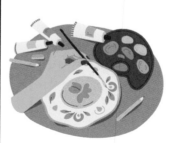 Crafting
Help	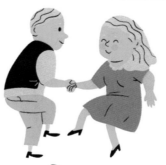 Dance	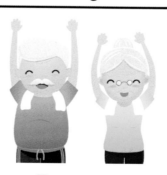 Exercise	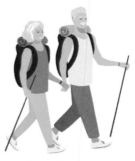 Outings
Done			

Activities

I want	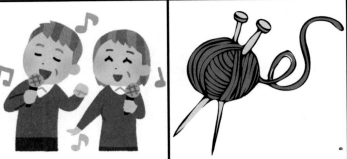 Singing	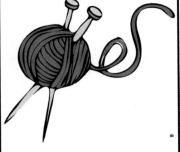 Knitting	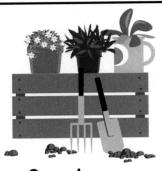 Gardening

I want

You

No

Change

More

Help

Done

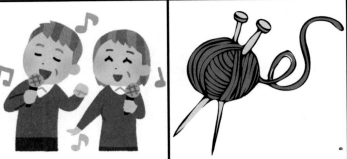	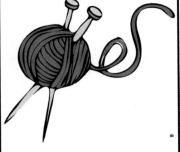	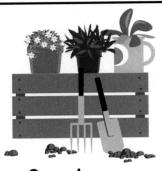
Singing	Knitting	Gardening
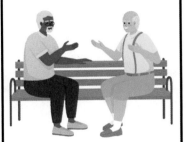	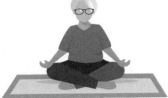	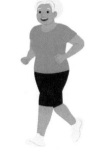
Companion	Meditation	Jogging
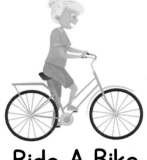	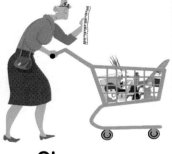	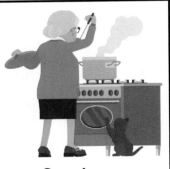
Ride A Bike	Shopping	Cooking

Places

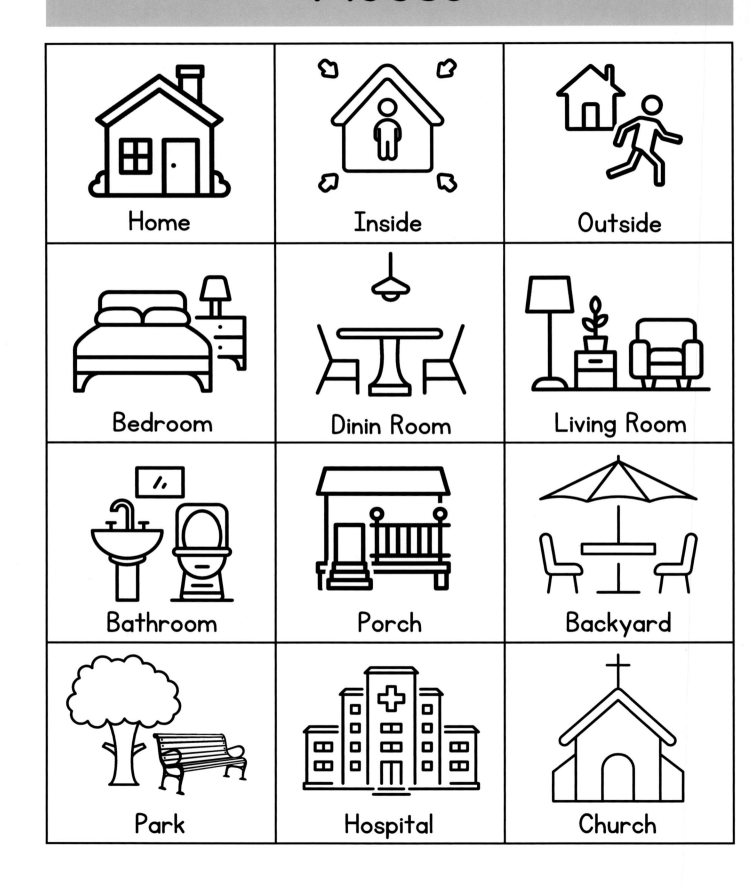

Home	Inside	Outside
Bedroom	Dinin Room	Living Room
Bathroom	Porch	Backyard
Park	Hospital	Church

Needs

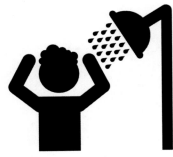Take a shower	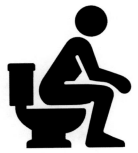Use Toilet	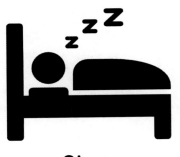Sleep
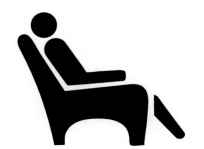Rest	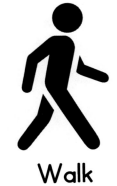Walk	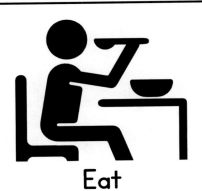Eat
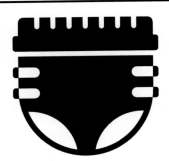Get Dressed	Change Diaper	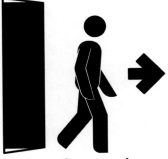Go Outside
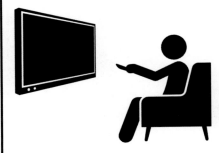Watch TV	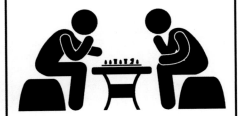Play	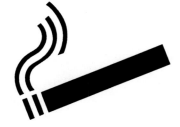Smoke

Needs

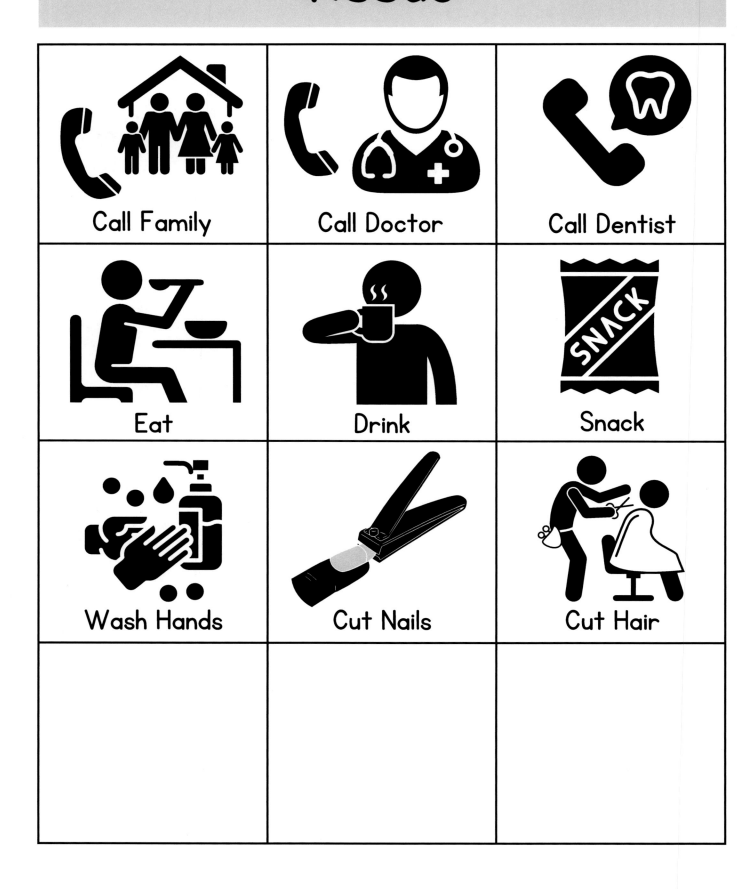

Call Family	Call Doctor	Call Dentist
Eat	Drink	Snack
Wash Hands	Cut Nails	Cut Hair

Items

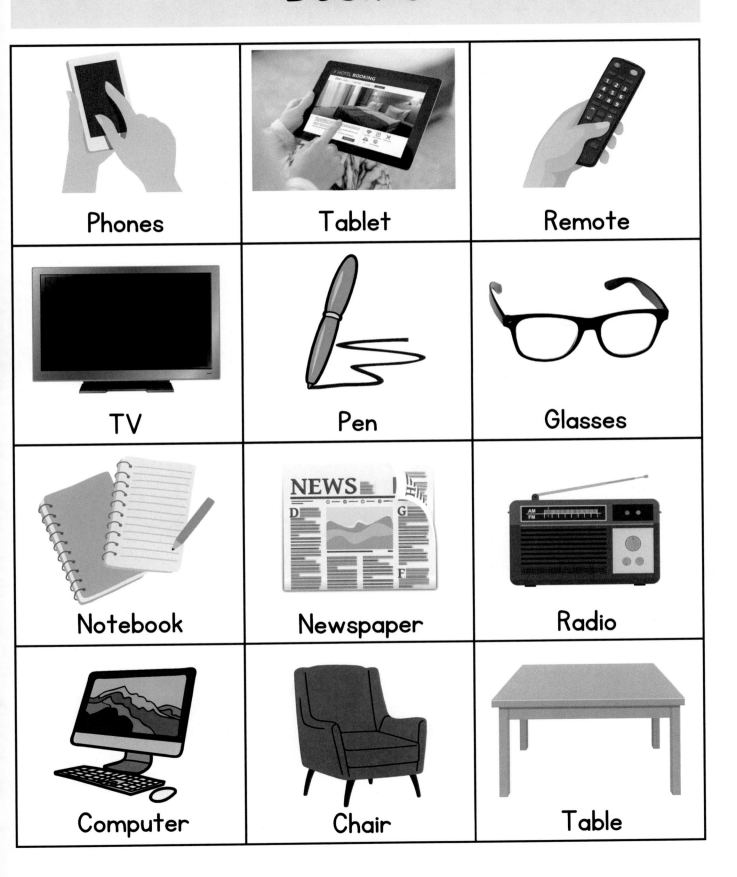

Phones	Tablet	Remote
TV	Pen	Glasses
Notebook	Newspaper	Radio
Computer	Chair	Table

Items

Add your own pictures here

Add your own pictures here

I need

You

No

Change

More

Help

Done

I need

You

No

Change

More

Help

Done

Add your own pictures here

Made in the USA
Las Vegas, NV
01 December 2024

13053780R00017